M000217720

NAVIGATING
ALZHEIMER'S

NAVIGATING
ALZHEIMER'S

12 Truths about Caring for Your Loved One

MARY K. DOYLE

in extenso

NAVIGATING ALZHEIMER'S
12 Truths about Caring for Your Loved One
by Mary K. Doyle

Edited by Michael Coyne
Design and typesetting by Patricia A. Lynch
Cover photo by Bigstock

Copyright © 2018 by Mary K. Doyle

Published by In Extenso Press
Distributed exclusively by ACTA Publications, 4848 N. Clark Street,
Chicago, IL 60640, (800) 397-2282, www.actapublications.com

All rights reserved. No part of this publication may be reproduced or
transmitted in any form or by any means, electronic, digital, or mechani-
cal, including photocopying and recording, or by any information storage
and retrieval system, including the Internet, without permission from the
publisher. Permission is hereby given to use short excerpts with proper cita-
tion in reviews and marketing copy, newsletters, bulletins, class handouts,
and scholarly papers.

Library of Congress Catalog Number: 2015932290
ISBN: 978-0-87946-989-4
Printed in the United States of America by Total Printing Systems
Year 25 24 23 22 21 20 19 18
Printing 12 11 10 9 8 7 6 5 4 3

♻ Text printed on 30% post-consumer recycled paper

Contents

Like sunshine
on an overcast day,
rays of the man I knew
peek through the clouds
leaving me longing for more.

Foreword by Herbert Sohn, MD

At last we have a book that will be truly valuable for anyone taking on the task of providing primary care to an individual with Alzheimer's disease.

Mary Doyle is not only an excellent writer but also has had tremendous experience taking care of her husband with Alzheimer's for many years. Being able to put such practical experience into language medical lay people can easily grasp is an art, and she has certainly perfected that art.

Her book not only explains the unique problems connected with the disease but also gives the reader real insights into what can be done to help both the individuals suffering from the disease and their volunteer caregivers.

It has been known for many years that one of the major causes of depression among people who take care of loved ones with Alzheimer's is that they are not prepared for the type and amount of work involved. Mary Doyle has given them a superb guide, and I congratulate her on the excellence of her endeavor.

Dr. Herbert Sohn is a member of the board of directors of Healing Our Veterans, which works with veterans with Alzheimer's, PTSD, and effects of strokes. His credentials include FACS (Fellow of the American College of Surgeons) and FACLM (Fellow of the American College of Legal Medicine). Dr. Sohn is a Past President of the American Association of Clinical Urologists and Past Vice-Chair of the Board of Trustees, University of Health Sciences, Chicago Medical School (now Rosalind Franklin University). He is also an attorney and a urologist in practice for over 50 years.

Setting Sail for the High Seas

Early in the disease, when I told someone that my husband had Alzheimer's, I got that deer-in-the-headlights look, the one that signals something terrible is about to happen and there is nothing you can do to stop it. There was no hiding their concern and sorrow for what we were about to face.

Caring for a loved one with Alzheimer's is like navigating a voyage on the high seas. The course offers an unpredictable combination of magnificent and turbulent experiences. Caregiver survival depends on steady footing, dependable support, and a lot of prayer.

As primary caregivers to someone with Alzheimer's, our responsibilities are at their maximum. Our undivided attention is needed every second of every day. Our loved ones' physical, emotional, and mental needs are in our hands. Unlike caring for children, who also require undivided attention, the journey of Alzheimer's is one of decline rather than growth, increasing dependence rather than independence. We must think for our loved ones in every way, and we realize that care will extend for the rest of their lives here on earth. Such intense care is wearing on our emotional and physical health as few other caregiving roles are.

But there is so much more to our experience than this. We also encounter grace-filled moments. The woman before us is the mother who nurtured, worried about, and prayed for us. This is the sibling we shared secrets with, the husband who was "our everything." Even in the late stages of our loved ones' Alzheimer's, we caregivers experience fragments of the person we knew. We hear stories from the past that we've long forgotten, or never heard, and share tender, loving moments meant only for us.

The care required is intimate and soulful. It's heart-wrenching and heart-warming. People with Alzheimer's are often agitated, frustrated, and confused. But they also can be quite sweet, innocent, and profoundly appreciative of our presence.

My intention for this book is to offer solid information, understanding, compassion, and resources. Each chapter begins with a title/statement, an example of what that statement looks like in action, and what I learned from that aspect of caring for someone with Alzheimer's. Most chapters include bullet points and each ends with a short list of practical suggestions.

I have no medical background. I am a professional writer with a Master's Degree in Pastoral Theology. I write from experience. My husband, Marshall, has Alzheimer's. I cared for him myself at home for the first nine years of his illness, called in caregiving assistance the tenth year, and I have now moved him to an assisted living home exclusively for memory care.

Our situation is different than most because Marshall was an entertainer his entire adult life. In some ways his past profession makes the journey easier. In other ways it makes it more difficult.

Marshall, at least at this point, doesn't have the fear of strangers most people with Alzheimer's do. For them, when they walk into a room of people they do not know it is as if they were transplanted to another country where nothing is familiar. In contrast, Marshall often assumes these strangers are fans and so is less frightened of them than he might be otherwise. Being center stage is familiar to him, something few people with Alzheimer's feel.

Marshall can't hold much of a conversation anymore, but he has performed magic since he was a child and still can do some tricks. His playful manner and magic skills continue to spark laughter in the people around him. This allows him to connect with others in a meaningful and positive way.

Our large family and a small circle of friends see him often, but we ask that others, beyond those closest to him, respect his privacy. It is best for his health and safety that fans and other more casual friends do not visit. He loved and appreciated them all, but at this time the visits are too wearing on him.

Basically, though, our story is similar to most. Sprinkles of our personal experiences are scattered throughout this book. I share these moments when I think they offer something for you to relate to. If nothing else, I hope they demonstrate that you are not alone.

I encourage you to call on family, friends, your church or congregation, and public agencies for help. We caregivers of those with Alzheimer's cannot, and need not, do it alone. It truly takes a village to care for someone with Alzheimer's. There are an estimated 5.5 million Americans living with dementia due to Alzheimer's, and each person requires at least three to five people to care for them. Additionally, only one in four with Alzheimer's are believed to have been diagnosed. So, the number of people necessary to provide care for all our loved ones is extensive.

Reach out to other caregivers. Talk with people who know what you are going through. You will find a list of organizations in the resource section of this book that can help you find support groups.

Marshall's outstanding neurologist calls Alzheimer's "The caregivers disease" because it is so exhausting for the loving friends and family who care for those with Alzheimer's, often for years or even decades. In addition, often when one family member— a spouse, one of the children, or a close friend—is the primary caregiver, it can result in anger and resentment, power struggles, changes in dynamics of relationships, and loss of the caregiver's own independence. For these reasons, the illness necessitates that we caregivers count on other people to assist us as we assist our loved ones. It forces us to acknowledge that we human beings need one another and truly are all connected, one person to the next.

1. Alzheimer's Is Not a Part of Normal Aging

WHAT IT'S LIKE

Your husband went out to run some routine errands and said he would be back in an hour. Four hours later he calls from a clerk's phone at a convenience store across town. He doesn't know where he's been or where he is. This is not the first time, and it will surely not be the last.

WHAT I LEARNED

If we suspect something is wrong with a loved one's memory, we need to arrange a medical evaluation right away. They will be reluctant to go, but early intervention can make a significant difference in how things progress from then on.

We are our brother's keeper, and this statement is never truer than when someone we love has Alzheimer's. We are their advocate, guardian, caregiver, and friend, and successfully filling these roles is vitally important—from the first suspicions of the disease.

At first we know something is wrong, but we don't know exactly what it is. Our mother seems more distracted, forgetful, agitated, and confused. She is short-tempered and argumentative. She may even be sexually inappropriate. Basically, she just doesn't act like the person we knew. We wonder if it is normal aging or an indication that something has changed in our relationship or in her health. Our worst fear is that it has something to do with her loss of memory or, even worse, an early sign of Alzheimer's.

The suspicion of any memory disease is terrifying. So many parts of our relationship are threatened. Not only is the present day in jeopardy, but our entire future with them is too. Where do we even start to find answers? Whom do we turn to for help?

We begin by considering the type and extent of symptoms we are noticing. Some physical illnesses can manifest changes in personality as much as mental illnesses do. When we do not feel well it takes a toll on our emotional and mental well-being too. Initially, it may be difficult to discern if this is merely a temporary condition or something more ominous.

We also need to analyze the extent of the memory issues. It's normal to occasionally forget a name, miss an appointment, misplace a cell phone, or forget to pay a bill. We all do these things, especially if we are busy, distracted, or constantly multi-tasking.

If these episodes are happening often, however, check with a physician. Our loved ones aren't likely to recognize the state of their current condition or openly admit to any deficit. They may minimize their problems out of fear and an understandable lack of objectivity. A good physical exam by an observant physician—especially one skilled in dealing with the elderly—can rule out common causes for temporary dementia, such as a thyroid imbalance, alcohol abuse, or conflict with a medication.

If there is no apparent cause, a basic memory screening will be given. Further testing may include brain scans, blood work to check biomarkers, and neuropsychological exams for a more accurate diagnosis. Newer tests, such as analyzing saliva, blood, or cerebral fluid, are helpful in forming a correct diagnosis, although the only way to absolutely confirm Alzheimer's disease at this point is by examining the brain after death.

In any event, although there is no known cure or irrefutable diagnosis, early intervention can help manage, and possibly slow, the progression of Alzheimer's symptoms. Nerve cells in the brain begin dying long before symptoms are noticeable, so the sooner treatment begins, the greater the efficacy of the long-term care for our loved ones and, ultimately, the better their quality of life—and, by extension, ours.

Even if we have long suspected that our loved ones do indeed have Alzheimer's, the final diagnosis of it is devastating. I clearly remember the day the doctors told our family that test results made it pretty clear that my husband, Marshall, had Alzheimer's disease. It had become more and more evident with each disappointing test result, but the words telling us that it was indeed true were painful to hear.

My body physically reacted to the news with a churning stomach and throbbing head. I wondered what that meant for us and our future as a family. I worried it was the end of our marriage as we knew it.

Alzheimer's certainly has changed the course of our relationship. We've met insurmountable challenges. You will too. But I guarantee you that you also will have warm, loving, and joyful times as well. You need only to keep your heart open (and get plenty of rest, which isn't easy to do if your loved one is up throughout the night).

If you suspect a problem with your loved one's memory, consider the differences between typical, age-related changes and budding signs of Alzheimer's:

DIFFERENCE BETWEEN NORMAL AGING AND ALZHEIMER'S	
Typical Age-Related Changes	Signs of Alzheimer's
Missing a payment	Inability to manage a budget or balance a checkbook
Not knowing an occasional date	Rarely or never knowing the date or not knowing the season.
Occasionally losing an item	Often losing things and not being able to retrace steps
Forgetting a name but remembering it later	Forgetting the names of grandchildren or other close family members
Occasionally making bad decisions	Inability to make a decision
Slower learning process	Inability to learn new skills and information
Confusing the remote with the phone	Not recognizing the phone for what it is

WHAT CAUSES ALZHEIMER'S?

Dementia refers to a group of symptoms that include mental confusion, memory loss, disorientation, intellectual impairment, inability to learn new things, and repetition. Alzheimer's disease is a particular form of dementia that typically manifests these types of symptoms and an array of others including depression, irritability, hallucinations, and paranoia. Initially, the change in personality may be more apparent than the memory loss. It often is what family members notice first.

Alzheimer's disease is the sixth leading cause of death in the U.S. Approximately 500,000 people die each year as a result of this disease. One in three seniors dies suffering from some form of dementia.

According to 2017 statistics, Alzheimer's affects 5.5 million Americans, and that number is expected to soar to 16 million by 2050. Most people with Alzheimer's are 65 years of age or older. The probability of developing it increases with age. The rate is higher in women, partly because women live longer.

Symptoms of Alzheimer's vary with a person's disposition, pre-existing health conditions, and the advancement of the disease. The disease is irreversible and progressive. The decline may transpire over a few years or may take decades. In advanced stages, assistance is needed with bathing, dressing, toileting, and eating. In the final stages, the ability to communicate and recognize loved ones is lost and the person with the disease requires continuous care.

There remains much that is unknown about Alzheimer's and its causes. It appears to result from a combination of genetic, lifestyle, and environmental factors. Suspected risk factors include depression, high cholesterol, Type 2 diabetes, high blood pressure, and excessive weight. New studies suggest a deficiency in Vitamin

D and hearing loss may be contributing factors, and head injuries may also play a role.

The risk of developing the disease is somewhat higher if a parent or sibling has it now or had it in the past. There are mutations in three genes that increase the likelihood of getting Alzheimer's by about 5 percent. The strongest risk gene known at this time is apolipoprotein e4 (APOE e4).

The occurrence of Alzheimer's appears less often in people with higher levels of formal education. A stimulating job, mentally challenging leisure activities like reading, frequent social interactions, playing a musical instrument, and even just playing games or doing crossword puzzles may all help to prevent Alzheimer's. Studies show that healthy eating, brain and physical activity, and good heart health may slow dementia for people at risk for the disease.

Alzheimer's is believed to manifest in what are called "plaques and tangles" throughout the cortex of the brain. Plaque consists of protein fragments called beta-amyloid that build up between nerve cells. Tangles are twisted fibers of a protein called "tau" that accumulate inside cells. Both plaques and tangles destroy the ability of nerve cells to function and communicate.

From the mid-stages of Alzheimer's on, a loved one will require 24/7 attention. Supervision and cueing (prompting) are needed to keep them safe and on track. They may be able to do quite a bit for themselves for many years, as long as someone is nearby to guide them.

Some treatments and therapies are thought to help with the symptoms, making life easier for both the person with the disease and their caregivers. Medications may lessen the severity of symptoms, for at least a limited time. Behavior modification is often also effective.

Behavior modification involves changing the way a person responds to stimulus. It uses positive reinforcement, opportunities to excel, and the process of redirecting a loved one stuck on a particular thought to prevent their agitation or insistence on something from escalating.

From the time of diagnosis, I made an effort to protect Marshall's dignity and keep him socially and physically active. I closely monitored his medications, supplements, and diet. I continued to treat him respectfully as an adult, my husband, and a senior 20 years older than I am. Our doctors believe my actions contributed significantly in delaying the pace of his further deterioration. The extra effort on my part benefited him, me, and our relationship for many years.

....

THREE THINGS TO DO
AS SOON AS YOU SUSPECT DEMENTIA

1. Don't delay talking to your physician.

2. Rule out other physical illnesses. Screen for Alzheimer's and other forms of dementia.

3. Seek ongoing neuropsychological care.

....

2. The Manner and Length of Illness Cannot Be Predicted

WHAT IT'S LIKE

You love your little home in Arizona, but wonder
if it is time to move back up north, close to your
children, who can help you care for your husband.
You'd like to know when you should put your
house on the market and start packing. If you knew
how long it will be before you will be unable to
care for him alone, your decision would be so much
easier.

WHAT I LEARNED

No one knows exactly what will happen in the
future, the specific manner in which the disease
will progress, or how long our loved ones will live.
Our best option is to suppress worrying, to remain
present, and enjoy what we do have.

We all have an inherent need to know what to expect in the future, but especially when it comes to health, no one can fully give us the answers we so desperately seek. Doctors can offer a reasonable prognosis based on their education, expertise, and experience, but there's no crystal ball to predict the exact path of the illness.

When my mother was diagnosed with cancer, her physician told me that he expected that she only had about six more weeks to live. My mother (and the Lord) didn't agree. She lived another three years.

My friend Marlene described another example. Her mother had advanced Alzheimer's disease and refused to eat. Doctors inserted a feeding tube. They warned the family she was near death.

Two years later the skin surrounding the tube became inflamed and the tube fell out. Desperate to assure that she received nourishment, Marlene and her father tried to feed her mother some soft food by mouth. To their surprise her mother swallowed the food and continued eating by mouth for the next three years.

The National Alzheimer's Association predicts that Alzheimer's can last anywhere from three to twenty years, with an average time span of about eight years. This wide span offers us little help in predicting how much remaining time we have with our loved ones. There are so many variables to consider that the full prognosis of any one case is impossible to predict. A person's age, current overall health, other preexisting conditions and diseases, mental outlook, support system—and ultimately, God's will—control the outcome. No one can tell us exactly what will happen when.

The elusive unknown makes planning a future with a loved one with Alzheimer's challenging. Throughout my husband Marshall's disease, I've had many questions. I've wanted to know what was next, how long he would know me, how long could I care for him myself, what will happen in the end, and how much time we have left together.

When I told his first neuropsychologist that I'd read that people with Alzheimer's could live twenty years with the disease, she said that even ten more years was unrealistic for Marshall. She estimated he could have as many as five or as few as one or two more years.

Marshall has shown symptoms of Alzheimer's disease severe enough to disrupt daily life since at least 2004. At this writing, although confused with little short-term memory and physically declining as well, he is outliving many of his apparently healthy peers the same age.

For others, the opposite is true. They have much less time than expected. Some families barely have an opportunity to say good-bye. Their loved one's illness progresses like wildfire.

We can't anticipate the course of the disease any more than the length. Educating ourselves on the illness can help us understand symptoms as we encounter them and hint at what's likely to be ahead. Established guidelines for what we may expect are often grouped into stages with symptoms common for each. But again, everyone is different and has a variety of other conditions to consider. No one's journey through Alzheimer's is identical to anyone else's. The health story changes when we mix hypertension, diabetes, and other illnesses with Alzheimer's, as well as the unique workings of our own bodies.

If you are like me, understanding the disease more fully will help you feel better prepared for what might happen, lessening your worries. To learn more about Alzheimer's:

- Sign up for newsletters from dependable websites like alz.org and mayoclinic.com.

- Send for brochures from the Alzheimer's Association.

- Ask for resources from your local facilities for people with Alzheimer's.

- Join support groups at the nearest hospital.

- Talk with other families who care for loved ones with Alzheimer's.

- Inquire which local, county, and state agencies may be of service.

In spite of his illness, Marshall and I have had many good years and I am certain will continue to have wonderful moments ahead. As much as the family would like to know how and when the story will end, we can't; so we might as well focus on the treasures of the day and remain in the present moment as much as possible.

Although Marshall knows he has the disease, like most people with Alzheimer's, he has never been aware of the extent of his disability. He believes there is little hindering his daily functions. Because I am fully aware of his limitations, I've made a conscious effort not to allow anything to interfere with our gentle, loving relationship. I appreciate every little hug, smile, and "I love you." I'm acutely aware that even these gifts will cease soon enough.

Marshall's neurologist gave us sound advice at the time of diagnosis: Don't anticipate or worry about what might happen. Every person has a unique physical and emotional history and, therefore, the way the disease will develop is unpredictable. Handle each issue as it arises rather than worry about problems that may never occur. And remember, stay positive. New advances in medicine are always happening. A cure may be right around the corner.

WHAT TO DO ABOUT THE FUTURE

1. Do not become overly concerned about what might happen. Worrying about tomorrow's imaginary problems will solve nothing and can diminish our appreciation of the very real, unfolding present.

2. Handle each situation as it comes.

3. Remain positive and hopeful.

3. People with Alzheimer's Have at Least Two Different Personalities

WHAT IT'S LIKE

You had a lovely day with your mother. You took her to the doctor, where things went well, and to lunch, where she enjoyed one of her favorite dishes. She spoke with enthusiasm and apparent clarity about the present and the past. But later in the day, as the sun set, she became agitated and confused. She reached a point where she didn't fully recognize you and demanded that you leave her apartment immediately.

WHAT I LEARNED

Our loved ones are always present but not always visible. They may seem like our parents one minute and strangers the next. We must try not to take their words and actions personally. They have no control over them. We do have control over ours.

A change in personality is often the first indication of Alzheimer's disease. You may notice that your mother is more irritable than she used to be. The mood swings will continue as the disease progresses. As simple daily tasks become more challenging for her, she will feel and act like a frustrated toddler. Planning and preparing meals, planting flowers, or managing her finances may pose insurmountable problems for her. She momentarily knows what she wants to do but can't seem to follow through with the task and then forgets altogether what she was doing. If you are with her when she is agitated, she's likely to project her frustration on you.

Your mother no longer can separate fact from fiction, past from present, or reality from fantasy. Everything is jumbled as in a dream-like state. Her perception of the world is distorted. Information comes out like puzzle pieces disconnected and senseless on their own. This can be very upsetting and embarrassing for her if she is aware of her inability to function as fully as she used to.

The Alzheimer's sufferer's brain deteriorates and his or her memories are lost in the reverse order in which they were acquired. Most recent information is typically the first to go. It is like a movie on the old VHS tape in rewind, but with parts completely missing. Only some fragments of each period remain, scrambled and indecipherable. Place this condition in the midst of today's stressful and sensory-overloaded environment and it's understandable why people with Alzheimer's struggle to process it all.

Sometimes their limitations aren't as apparent as at others. One day your mother may identify her surroundings and the things and people around her with ease. The next day she may not. She is suddenly frightened and follows you from room to room like a child.

Her emotions will fluctuate as well. You see her fade in and out through the day and night and, as the disease progresses, the balance of those symptomatic times continue to move inexorably in the Alzheimer direction. She will more often be confused than not, and unless controlled with medication her unpredictability makes it increasingly difficult for you to relate to her.

A friend described her relationship with her mother like this:

> *When the first signs of Alzheimer's started popping up, my mother was "in" more than "out." She was not forgetting names, repeating ideas, or showing noticeable personality changes. She was the mother I knew. As the disease progressed, things started to shift. There were more and more times of "out," which included forgetfulness, mood changes, repeating, etc.*
>
> *Then, there were years when it was 50/50. She knew me as often as she did not. During this time my father and I remained in denial about the disease. We didn't want to see what was happening.*
>
> *In the final stages, she was almost entirely "out." There were only brief periods of recognition. The one time late in the disease when she called me by name, it was a surprise and delight to all who were around.*

Whether they are "in" or "out" will affect how our loved ones reacts to us. A hug from a woman's husband is comforting. But if she thinks the man is a stranger, that hug will be frightening. Taking extra care to look at life from their perspective, seeing things through their eyes instead of our own, can help us better understand where they are coming from.

This constant giving and withdrawal of their love will set

most of us on an emotional roller coaster. One day a husband tells his wife that she is the love of his life, that she means everything to him. A day later he does not even know they are married. The wife who has dedicated decades of her life to caring for him is now a stranger. Understanding that he has no control over his thoughts makes her feel no less sad.

While we are in a relationship with someone with Alzheimer's disease, it feels as if we are dealing with two different people. When our loved ones are lucid, we can engage in a basic conversation. Things run fairly smoothly. We'll even enjoy sweet moments together. When our loved ones become agitated, or confused, or repeat the same statement over and over and over and over again, it is exhausting.

A common condition for people with Alzheimer's disease, known as "sundowning," is one of the many reasons for that difference in personality. The syndrome is a mood and behavior change that occurs later in the day. It is also noticeable, inexplicably, when the barometer falls.

The causes of sundowning are not well understood. Overstimulation and fatigue, disorientation stemming from the inability to separate dreams from reality, confusion over shadows, the onset of darkness, hormonal imbalances, and an upset in the internal body clock may all contribute.

There are a few simple things we can do to minimize sundowning, but we can't expect to totally suppress it. Best practices include ensuring our loved ones have a structured day that includes exercise, maintaining a calm home with plenty of light in the house, avoiding sugars, alcohol, and caffeine, and discouraging lengthy naps. However, some people do better with a short, structured afternoon rest followed by a favorite activity to encourage them to get up and continue with the rest of their day. While these things can be helpful, they will not solve all the behavior issues.

We also must be mindful of other medical problems that can aggravate symptoms. People with Alzheimer's cannot always express what is wrong with them in ways we easily understand. They may not feel well but may be unable to tell us anything is wrong.

Wandering may or may not be related to sundowners, but it is another important concern. We may not need to be with our loved ones every second, but we do need to know what they are doing and where they are at all times, especially if they have demonstrated a tendency to wander. While not all people with Alzheimer's wander, the potential danger is so great that the possibility cannot be ignored. While it may occur at any time, it is most common after a move or when they are restless, agitated, or bored.

Increased physical activity helps to curb both sundowning and wandering. We also should have some reasonable safety measures in place. This includes installing a baby monitor in a loved one's room, a security system in the house, and safety locks on all doors. It also is important for our loved ones to wear identification bracelets. If your loved one carries a wallet, be sure the wallet contains a current photo ID and your own contact information. In addition, your wallet should contain a slip of paper stating, "In case of emergency please note that if my well-being is in jeopardy and my loved one is with me, call this number immediately. My loved one has Alzheimer's disease and is not capable of caring for themselves even if they insist that they are."

Keeping our loved ones safe requires us to make many difficult decisions. It is our responsibility to ensure their well-being, even if many of our actions deprive them of the things in life that give them personal satisfaction. While we do not want to restrict their rights and privileges, we often must for their own welfare.

For years I watched my husband Marshall's driving abilities decline. He'd always been the main driver and enjoyed cars and driving. He was a poor passenger. He liked to be in control. I dreaded taking the car away from him and put it off much longer than I should have. It wasn't until we'd taken a long drive with my stepson, who pointed out how unsafe his dad's driving was— not just for us but for everyone on the road—that I knew I could wait no longer.

Marshall was angry at the very beginning but, surprisingly, didn't say much about it after the thought settled. We sold his car, which seemed to help him get a better grasp of the situation. For the most part, he accepted that I was his driver, willing to take him wherever he wanted to go. The situation taught me an important lesson: delaying a necessary change because I did not want to hurt Marshall's feelings was pointless, irresponsible, and potentially dangerous.

It's one of the many decisions we cannot avoid making on our loved ones' behalf. Here are a few others commonly encountered while caring for someone with Alzheimer's, and some basic guidelines to help decide when to take action:

When is it time to:

- **Go to the doctor?** As soon as we suspect problems with memory, we must see our physician. If results are inconclusive but symptoms continue or worsen, we should go back to the doctor or get another opinion.

- **Take over the finances?** When bills are paid late or not at all, money is lost or randomly given away, or the checkbook cannot be balanced, finances should be handled by a trusted family member.

- **Take the car keys?** When reaction time or motor skills are impaired, when decision-making falters, if they are easily distracted, confused as to their whereabouts, or have difficulty following directions, the car keys need to be retrieved. It's far better to prevent driving before a serious accident than after one.

- **Call in additional help?** Hire caregivers with memory care experience, or enlist trusted friends and family, to alternate care with us as soon as a diagnosis is made. For our own sake as a caregiver, and for the sake of our loved ones, *we must not delay* recruiting assistance.

- **Take personal time?** Scheduled weekly days off and a regular vacation break from providing care should be taken by primary caregivers from the time of diagnosis to prevent burn-out. It can be difficult to give ourselves permission to do this. But it is critical for our own health and ability to maintain our stamina. Alzheimer's is not a puddle jump. It is an ocean voyage.

- **Have someone with our loved ones at all times?** When they've had incidences concerning safety, fear, or wandering, they should no longer be left home alone.

- **Place our loved ones in a memory-care home?** They should be moved to a memory-care home when our own home is no longer safe or healthy for us or for them. As the disease progresses, one caregiver cannot possibly do everything alone. Our loved ones will eventually need a coordinated and experienced team wherever they reside.

- **See an attorney?** Right now! Important documents—including a will and a medical power of attorney—should be in place long before they are required.

Because of the difficulty of these decisions, we naturally tend to delay taking action longer than we should. We don't want to hurt our loved ones' feelings, but our responsibility to keep them safe is far more important. These are times when we have to rely on our heads, not our hearts, and find the courage to do what we know we need to do.

WHAT TO DO WHEN YOU OBSERVE TWO DIFFERENT PERSONALITIES

1. Enjoy the good moments.

2. Realize it's all part of the illness.

3. Work through the tough times as calmly as possible.

---

4. We Play an Important Role in Our Loved Ones' Behavior

WHAT IT'S LIKE

Your father, now living with you and spending most of his days alone in his room, storms down the stairs and accuses you of taking money from his wallet. You insist you'd never do that. The argument escalates and he becomes increasingly agitated. You are hurt, defensive, and argue back. Before long, he no longer remembers what the argument is about but is raging out of control.

WHAT I LEARNED

When we caregivers find our loved ones becoming agitated, we are the ones who need to calm down. Our loved ones will reflect our mood and reactions, and the situation will get better for all of us if we can remain peaceful and positive.

Like it or not, we are responsible for some of our loved ones' temperament. They mirror our moods. If we are frustrated or irritable, most likely our loved ones will become so also. Alzheimer's sufferers certainly can be difficult, repetitive, and agitated. And we certainly can become tired and overwhelmed with the amount of work we need to do. But it is imperative that we remain calm. There's no guarantee that maintaining our composure will keep them from being agitated, and staying calm may be extremely challenging, but it can prevent a situation from getting out of hand. If we remain positive, they have a far better chance of remaining positive, or returning to a positive frame of mind.

Some typical symptoms of Alzheimer's are more troubling than others. The repetition of words and actions that is so common among sufferers is difficult to ignore. Our parent or spouse asks a question that requires a basic response, and we answer. But sometimes the spinning cycle of endless repetition of the same question or statement is as irritating as fingernails grating on a chalkboard.

"Why can't you take me with you?" or "I don't like this food," when said countless times in succession, feel like judgment or criticism. They have no idea their remarks are hurtful to hear or that they are wearing our emotions thin. In their minds, they are voicing their opinion or request only once.

Our response must be one of compassion and respect, difficult as that can be. We cannot correct them as we would a child, telling them to "be quiet" or "sit still," for example. They are adults and deserve to be treated with dignity.

This is a time when we need to divert our loved ones' attention. We might try changing the subject or responding in a different way. We can encourage them to participate in another activity and become interested in something else long enough to forget where they were stuck.

If that fails after several attempts, we may protect our own sanity by distracting ourselves with another activity. Pray or listen to soft music. Or turn up your loved one's favorite music. Music is a powerful tool. Familiar songs may relax everyone.

Obsessive and compulsive behaviors often parallel or accompany verbal repetition. They may blow their nose, wash their hands, or scratch themselves until they are raw. This may continue over a period of days or even years. Such behaviors may even harm them and need to be controlled with redirection or medication.

Other obsessions are more curious than harmful. One man I know owned several businesses, and in the midst of Alzheimer's was fixated on all the bills he thought he had to pay. He carried a brief case and peered endlessly over stacks of papers, jotting little numbers and notes in the margins. Day after day he worried about bills he no longer had to pay.

My Grandma Rose loved a party in her younger years. After an extensive series of TIAs (Transient Ischemic Attack—a disruption of blood flow to the brain, often referred to as mini-strokes), she developed dementia. She became suspended in bliss, thinking she was on her way to a big event. She'd happily comb her hair in anticipation. Even if it was a compulsion, it didn't really harm her or bother any of her family members.

These obsessions offer each of us a reason to examine where we ourselves concentrate our daily thoughts. Perhaps if we focus on what makes us happy the rest of our lives and later develop a dementia, we too will be stuck in "a happy place" like my grandmother.

Hurtful remarks, accusations, and paranoia are also common in people with Alzheimer's. We caregivers are working hard to provide compassionate care, but then they say we took something or harmed them in some way, no matter how much we try to assure them otherwise, they are not convinced and may become more agitated.

Even after we show them proof that we didn't do what they are accusing us of, they often continue to believe we did something wrong. Our instincts are to defend ourselves, but we cannot do that with someone with Alzheimer's. It will only result in an argument that makes absolutely no sense, leaving both sides angry. As difficult as it is, we are better off when we just let their accusations go.

No doubt, there will be embarrassing public scenes as well. You are out at a restaurant and Dad goes into a tirade when you leave more than a two-dollar tip, which was appropriate back in the 1940s. He accuses you of being wasteful and points out that today's tip is more than a meal cost back then. Of course it appears ludicrous to him.

Since time is a concept lost to people with Alzheimer's, it's not unusual for them to remark that we never come to see them or stay with them long enough when, in fact, we do. Our absences feel so much longer to them than they are. The natural response to this criticism is to defend ourselves, but doing so only fuels their anger. Our loved ones have little understanding of our world. Once we are out of sight, they don't remember us even being there. Our insistence that we just visited only frustrates them. All we can do in this case is acknowledge that we miss them too when we are away. We also may add that we are happy to see them now.

We cannot reason with our loved ones at this point. It is in our nature to correct them, try to change their behavior, or get them to understand what they are doing, but it's not likely they can do so. Telling them that something does not belong to them, arguing with them to take a shower when they insist they already did, or demanding that they cannot go out in their underwear, doesn't get us anywhere.

We have to agree, redirect, or simply listen. Most of all, we can't take their hurtful remarks personally. They can't help how they feel any more than we can. However, unlike them, we do have the ability to understand the situation and accept the way things are, whether we like it or not.

Again, we are the ones who have to change and go along for the ride. We have to let go of our personal pain and think clearly and unemotionally. Remember that our loved ones' sense of observation and reasoning is off. They really can't help perceiving things as they do. We are the only person in the relationship who can think clearly and make a decision that will defuse a crisis.

Simplifying as much in our lives as possible will help to relieve stress for loved ones and caregivers. Establishing simplicity as a mode of living is an important step in maintaining a calm environment. If our home, daily routine, responsibilities, and expectations are simpler, everything will go more smoothly.

Here are a few ways to do this:

- Don't talk too loudly or quickly, or express multiple thoughts at once. Ask one question at a time and wait patiently for a response. If your loved one doesn't understand, say the same thing in a different way, but still simply.

- Physically slow down. Too much movement agitates our loved ones as they try to follow what we are doing.

- Simplify the home by removing clutter. Too many items on walls and shelves may be over-stimulating. It makes focusing on any one item difficult for them. Remove large groupings of vases and other decorative pieces scattered throughout the home. (This will also keep the chore of dusting down as well, which is a nice side benefit!)

- Remove throw rugs and other items on the floors to prevent tripping.

- Keep stairways clear and gate them if necessary.

- Have as many bills paid automatically as possible.

- Prepare meals that are fresh, healthy, and uncomplicated.

- Delegate responsibilities to other family members when possible. Ask for help with meal preparation, running errands, and caregiving on regularly designated days.

- Check with your pharmacy about medication management. This task is not only time-consuming but difficult for people with poor eyesight or dexterity. Your pharmacy may be able to sort meds into daily doses in advance.

Our conversations with our loved ones need to be simplified as well, but this does not mean speaking to them as if they were children. While the caregiving role feels parental, our loved ones are adults and deserve to be treated as such. We want to speak in normal but gentle tones and use short, clear sentences. We also need to learn how to ask or encourage them to do something rather than tell them they must do it.

And we have to be careful not to ask some questions we typically would in a normal conversation. Inquiring about what they did earlier that day, even if it was an important event, is frustrating because they aren't likely to be able to retrieve that information. We have to discipline ourselves to remain in the now by showing we are interested in what they are doing and want to know how they feel *right this moment*.

Little white lies are not only acceptable but often preferable to the truth. If our loved ones refuse to take necessary medications, call them vitamins. If they want to go outside in the bitter cold, say you will do so after lunch. A trip to a dreaded doctor can be described as a trip out shopping. If pushed, we really can stop at a store as well.

Guiding our loved ones into activities they are reluctant to engage in often calls for a little misdirection. If Mom doesn't like to bathe, turn on soft music and distract her with casual conversation while escorting her into the tub. If she says she isn't hungry, ask her to sit while *you* eat, and then place a plate of food she likes in front of her. Walk with her to the restroom at regular intervals to avoid accidents, and offer a snack when she is agitated to distract her. These strategies for better outcomes take some thought and advance planning, but they often prevent emotional outbursts and other serious problems.

Our goal must be to set our loved ones up for success, to give them opportunities to "help" where they can. Ask them to fold laundry or place the napkins around the table. If they feel productive and positive about themselves, they are more likely to be at peace. When they are at peace, we have a chance to be at peace too.

WHAT TO DO TO KEEP THINGS RUNNING SMOOTHLY

1. Reflect an image of joy and calm.

2. Keep things basic and uncomplicated.

3. If you find yourself losing control and are able to do so, give yourself a time out and step away.

5.　Plans Require Flexibility

....

WHAT IT'S LIKE

You were attending your granddaughter's graduation. She worked hard, and achieved so much, and you couldn't wait for the moment when she would cross the stage in cap and gown. You were happy and proud to be there until your wife grew restless and finally found herself overwhelmed by the crowd. She cried uncontrollably and begged you to take her home.

WHAT I LEARNED

Little on our to-do list is truly important. We need to be flexible and accept wherever the day takes us.

Our culture is one of appointments, errands, activities, work, and play, all crammed into 16 hours or less. We feel the need to fill the day, and the only way to do as much as we want is to closely schedule everything.

This jam-packed day, however, does not allow the flexibility necessary for a sudden change in plans. When we have to rearrange multiple appointments, the most carefully considered schedule can topple to the ground. This can be extremely frustrating.

Know that when dealing with people with Alzheimer's, plans have to allow for delays, rescheduling, and cancelations. Rushing causes agitation and creates an environment of failure. Our loved ones move slowly, and sometimes not at all, so appointments need to be well spaced and flexible. It is more difficult for someone with Alzheimer's to perform well when under stress. And we become stressed when they are stressed.

Rather than feeling overwhelmed by all we feel we have to do, we can follow the Alcoholics Anonymous saying, "Just do the next right thing." Living one moment at a time, taking one step at a time, and handling one situation at a time is a manageable practice.

This means that our expectations must be limited. If we are able to attend activities of our choice, they will be few and far between. They also may have to be shortened or canceled at some point.

Before making a commitment, consider the following suggestions:

- Schedule doctor appointments mid-morning to early afternoon, when your loved one is more alert.

- When responding to parties and special events, inform the host that you and your loved one may arrive late, leave early, or not be able to attend at all without further notice.

- Consider the number of people and amount of stimulation expected at an event before deciding to attend. Too much activity can be very stressful for people with Alzheimer's.

- Avoid attending events late in the day.

- Allow rest time before and after any event or travel.

- Accept that, even if you have someone covering for you, you may need to cancel your own appointments when your loved one really needs you.

In the early years of our marriage, I helped Marshall with his work. I wrote his letters and business material, planned our business trips and social events, remembered contact names, and made a point of getting to know his friends and colleagues. I also assisted him on and off stage during shows.

As the years passed, I assisted and cared for him increasingly, and in a more personal way. His schedule became my schedule. The majority of my day was now all about him. His needs required my undivided attention. After all, he couldn't do any of it for himself.

My ability to attend activities I was interested in grew slim. I put my own career and personal life on hold. I realized that his needs demanded someone's full attention, and I wanted to be that someone. I don't regret this in any way. We have had many wonderful times together, even in the midst of his decline, that can never be replaced.

The plan that does work when caring for someone with Alzheimer's is one that allows for simple regularity: a schedule that includes bathing, healthy meals, an exercise such as stretching or walking, light entertainment, and regular bedtimes. The predictability of it is reassuring and calming, both to our loved ones and to us.

....

WHAT TO DO ABOUT PLANNING EVENTS

1. Allow enough time for appointments so there is no need to rush.

2. Remember that crowds and noisy situations are stressful for people with Alzheimer's and make your decisions accordingly.

3. Allow a time of rest before and after an event for yourself and your loved one.

....

6. Alzheimer's Prompts Perpetual Mourning

....

WHAT IT'S LIKE

You are alone on the deck with your coffee. You used to sit there with your husband in the evening, enjoying the afterglow of a quiet meal together, watching the sunset, and talking with shared pleasure about the events of the day. Now he rarely has anything to say. Tonight he nodded off to sleep hours ago. You take a sip of coffee. It has grown cold in the cup.

....

WHAT I LEARNED

Little bits of the person we know and love, and our relationship with them, continue to disappear.

....

Alzheimer's is often referred to as the "Long Good-bye." Our parent, spouse, sibling, or friend fades away right before our eyes. We lose the intimacy, conversation, companionship, and friendship we grew so accustomed to, as their ability to learn new things slips away little by little. In the later stages, they lose physical abilities as well.

Alzheimer's prompts a perpetual mourning in caregivers because of this unstinting stream of loss. We just begin to recover from one loss, and another comes along. Sometimes losses occur gradually, and we adjust steadily as the changes gnaw away at what was ours. For example, you and your spouse might have played word games together until your spouse began struggling with spelling, reading, and writing. One day, he or she just couldn't play any game at all.

Other times a loss feels sudden because of its significance. The first time we have to make a critical decision and realize our lifelong go-to guy can't help is devastating. Discussing an important dilemma becomes impossible. He or she has little understanding of what we are talking about. We have other friends, but they aren't the ones we really want to talk to. It's painful to reflect and remember when things were different or, worse, to project ourselves into the future and fear the growing darkness that lies ahead.

The losses keep a steady pace with our loved ones' decline. Their illness may slowly diminish or make jumps in steps and then plateau for a while, until there is another devastating drop.

Navigating the emotional course of Alzheimer's and related dementias forces us to examine our relationship with our loved ones and the very meaning of life itself. And if we are the primary caregiver, our every thought, word, and action can be continually challenged by our loved ones. We will finally understand the meaning of Jesus' admonition about losing our life for his sake (Matthew 10:39). Caring for a loved one with dementia is an all-consuming responsibility. We really do have to consign our own thoughts, feelings, and dreams to the back burner.

As primary caregivers, we have to become accustomed to many additional personal losses. We lose our freedom when we come to a point when we no longer can leave our loved ones alone. We lose our privacy when we must call in others to help. We lose our personal space as things are rearranged for safety or to accommodate others staying in our home. Our free time is severely limited. There is little opportunity to play or relax. We lose friendships. We lose career opportunities, income, and savings.

Our own emotional health will suffer too. The role reversal of parent and child or the on-and-off recognition of a marital or sibling relationship, strains our own emotional stability. This ongoing emotional turmoil can send us repeatedly into the grieving process. It's not unusual to experience Elisabeth Kübler-Ross's universally recognized stages of grief:

- Denial—the inability to accept what is happening;

- Anger—at God, ourselves, our loved ones, and the situation;

- Bargaining—where we beg God, or a higher power, to make things right again if we do something in exchange;

- Depression—a deep sadness that makes it difficult for us to function; and

- Acceptance—embracing the realization that this is the new reality of our life.

These emotional expressions may not come in predictable order, and we can flip-flop back and forth among them. For days we may be angry at other members of the family who aren't there to help, angry at God, or angry that so much has been taken from us and our loved ones. Another day we might just be sad. Sadness can easily descend to the full depths of clinical depression.

We have a right to mourn. A need to mourn. But we should be careful not to sink into the murky depths of our own misery. The losses we experience are continuous, so we may find it difficult to rise from the depression. Feeding our heartache with overeating, drinking, drugs, gambling, or even an abundance of self-pity will only serve to drag us ever deeper down.

If we find ourselves headed in these directions, we must get help immediately. We can seek out friends and solid counseling to help us keep going, to help us remember the good stuff. It is necessary for us as caregivers to also care for and nurture ourselves, lest we become unable to care for our loved ones at all.

I know this from experience. I am by nature a happy, positive person, but have found myself deep in depression many times over our Alzheimer's years. As the lights continue to dim in my husband, it perpetuates a state of mourning in me. I'm deeply saddened as, little by little, I say good-bye to another part of our marriage and the man I married. Most of the time I keep a smile on my face, while inside my heart is breaking.

To offset this, I begin each day in prayer and end each day in thanksgiving. I spend time with my family and friends and soak in their strength, love, and support. Our survival as caregivers requires that we make this type of conscious effort to swim above the deep, churning waters of Alzheimer's.

Every day becomes a bit more challenging when caring for someone with Alzheimer's. Appreciating the gift of the present is important, because the present will likely change tomorrow. The saying that we don't miss what we've got until it's gone has never been more apparent. With Alzheimer's, some small thing we love is always coming to an end. We really do need to make an effort to become more mindful of what we still have in these unfolding moments, rather than dwell on what we once had, and have lost.

Remaining in the present is something commonly recommended when in conversation with people with Alzheimer's. The distant past lies in scattered pieces, recent events rarely become memories, and the future is not on their radar at all. Holding conversations exclusively about what is presently happening is challenging for most of us. Our discussions with family and friends typically center on something interesting we did in the past or sharing our excitement about something we are hoping to do. Concepts of past and future may be incomprehensible for people with Alzheimer's. We can't ask them what they did that morning or what they are planning on doing tomorrow. Doing so asks them to respond in ways they simply cannot.

Instead, we might ask how they are at this very minute. We comment on the beautiful day or tell them how good they look in that shirt, how the color brings out their blue eyes. We can talk about how happy we are to be with them. If they bring up experiences from the past, we can listen but respond uncritically, even if the details are mixed up—as they usually are.

Often, their comments make little sense initially, but there usually are a few bright shards of truth in them. We all draw on past experiences to make sense of what is currently happening. People with Alzheimer's do the same; it's just that often the dots don't obviously connect. What they are relating to doesn't seem to match up with what we are discussing.

Remarks they make often seem senseless, jumbled, or even shocking. The first time our loved one asks us who we are is painful beyond words. They will say things about our relationship that may be upsetting. It hurts when they forget we are their child or spouse or sibling. We no longer feel special in their lives.

It's hard to understand how they can forget how much we mean to them. But as the disease progresses, our loved one will lose all attachments to the past. And that includes us. We are bound by a history and memories that have vanished from their mind. But not ours.

Still, we continue to have them in our lives, to enjoy in a new and different way. They may think of us as a friend or distant relative and feel connected to us in some way only they can experience. Although it may not be the relationship we long for, it will always have elements of love.

WHAT TO DO WHEN MOURNING

1. Lean on faith, family, and friends.

2. Stay present. Learn to enjoy what you do have with your loved one.

3. Seek counseling, exercise, rest, and good nutrition for yourself, without guilt.

7.   We Are Only Human

WHAT IT'S LIKE

You climb into bed at the end of another long day
and wish you'd been more patient. You feel guilty.
You know that your mother can't help how she is.
You toss in bed, vowing to try harder tomorrow.

WHAT I LEARNED

We are human and have limitations. We cannot
complete all our responsibilities perfectly all the
time. We will have opportunities to do better
tomorrow.

Caring for someone with Alzheimer's can raise feelings of failure, guilt, and dishonesty in the caregiver. So much is asked of us that it is impossible to do everything perfectly; we can only do our best at the moment. When we fail, we can strive to do better the next time. When we succeed, we should pat ourselves on the back.

We often are forced to do things in the best interest of our loved ones that would feel distinctly wrong in any other situation. In an effort to avoid stress in them, we tell little lies, work around their back, and discuss their personal issues with professionals when they are out of earshot. We must place ourselves in the midst of their finances, health, and disabilities. It isn't what we want to do, but we must. We do it for them, but we don't feel good about it.

We will have to pay bills when our husband isn't around, grab the mail before he sees bills with his name on them—they never will get paid if he takes them—and have household repairs completed when he is not home to avoid his wanting to handle tools that have become dangerous.

There is a good deal of lying and avoidance of truth. If an activity is too stimulating for your mother, you tell her it was canceled. When she asks if her long-deceased brother is coming to visit, you respond, "Not today. He is busy."

And we blame the doctors for everything. We say, for example, that the doctor said they cannot fly any more or that it is the doctor who said we have to accompany them to the store. No doubt, the doctors really will help us with these things. If asked in advance, they really will tell your mother that she cannot drive, that they are taking away her driver's license. Mom won't remember a doctor telling her this, but from then on it will be a little easier for *us* to tell her that it was doctor's orders.

It isn't likely she will comprehend why she can't do something. Few people with Alzheimer's are aware of their cognitive decline. We cannot explain it to them. They do not think anything has changed.

When people have physical disabilities, they can easily grasp why they must do certain things for the good of their health. But with cognitive impairments, they rarely understand. There is no way to explain what has to be done. Our only way of coaxing them along is to say what is easiest for them to comprehend and what causes them the least amount of stress. The things we do to make them feel better make us feel worse.

It's not unusual for caregivers, especially family members, to feel guilty, but guilt accomplishes nothing. Author Jo Huey begins her book, *Alzheimer's Disease: Ten Simple Solutions for Caregivers*, with the statement that guilt is never helpful. She knows this is a common problem for caregivers and wants to help us eliminate those thoughts from our daily thinking. Huey advises us to acknowledge that we are doing the best we can, and let the rest go.

I'm quick to forgive others for their mistakes. I try to understand why they did what they did and see things from their point of view. For some reason, I'm highly intolerant of my own failings. It's difficult for me to forgive and forget my own shortcomings.

Yet, I know this is counterproductive. As a Christian, I believe God forgives me, and that should be all I need. I diminish my future effectiveness with my husband Marshall when I carry the burden of my past failings along the way. I have learned that little we caregivers do while caring for our loved ones is really failing.

We learn to care for them as we go. We aren't trained experts. We also are fallible. We are going to make mistakes, not have nearly enough patience, and experience days when we can't do anything right. Life is like that.

What we can do is continue to learn about the disease, strive to do better every day, and get enough rest. Everything is easier when we've had a good night's sleep. If we can't sleep at night, we need to sneak in a nap during the day. And we must remember to acknowledge to ourselves what we do well.

Take a minute and ask yourself:

- Am I doing what I can to keep my loved one safe?

- Am I monitoring my loved one's meals?

- Am I providing assistance with daily living such as bathing and toileting?

- Am I seeing to my loved one's medical needs?

- Am I providing my loved one with good care when I am not available?

- Am I seeing that my loved one's finances and other personal business are in order?

- Am I showing love and compassion to my loved one?

If we can honestly say we are doing our best with the short list above, we are already fulfilling a tall order. We don't have to do everything ourselves, but do have to see that things are done by someone competent to do so.

Caring for an Alzheimer's sufferer is one of the most challenging jobs possible, because there is so much to do, and dealing with someone who has no sense of reasoning puts a distinct and difficult twist on everything. Yet, here we are, putting one foot in front of the other, providing multi-level, compassionate care to someone we deeply love.

WHAT TO DO WHEN WE FEAR WE'VE FAILED

1. Vow to do better next time.

2. Forgive ourselves for telling the little white lies that make life easier for the one we love.

3. Take a break.

8. Outsiders Rarely Understand

WHAT IT LOOKS LIKE

A friend, trying her best to be encouraging, assures you, "Your mother looks great. She is so strong and healthy. You're lucky her symptoms aren't as bad as my neighbor's mom."

WHAT I LEARNED

People will say things, often with the best of intentions, that sting, upset and offend us. It will feel as if they are being willfully oblivious, insensitive, or critical. The truth is that it is difficult for anyone who has not experienced caring for someone with Alzheimer's to understand the overwhelming challenges confronting those of us going through it.

People peek inside a window to your home and think they know what it is like to live there. They talk about the other people they know with Alzheimer's disease. But spending an occasional afternoon with someone with the illness is nothing like bearing the responsibility of caring for them around the clock, hour after hour, day after day.

Thoughtless comments may even come from dear friends and family members, people we naturally feel should know better. It's hard to understand why they don't begin to fathom the depth of your loved one's disability or the confounding demands that are being made of you.

No doubt, their intention is not to be hurtful. In reality, they can't even begin to understand how stressful such caregiving is. Witnessing the symptoms of Alzheimer's in short time-frames is as different from providing continual care as running to the mailbox is from running a long-distance marathon.

You may hear apparently thoughtless remarks like:

- **He is so alert when we talk.** Outsiders are not aware that their brief conversation is a single moment of clarity, not the overall picture. A diagnosis of Alzheimer's does not mean all the lights are out, that our loved ones know nothing. Until the very last stages of the disease, our loved ones should be able to engage in casual conversation, especially if they are doing the talking or telling stories they enjoy. This is completely different from the give and take of an engaging, intellectual conversation, which becomes increasingly unlikely.

- **I know other people who are much more difficult to handle.** No one knows the challenges of caring for your loved one but you. No one else is there 24/7. No one else can possibly assess your situation with accuracy. As much as we may wish they might, it is unreasonable to expect that they will.

- **That's too late to be giving Dad his dinner.** Keeping pace with all that needs to be done in a day is difficult. Perhaps if the person who is making the comment became more aware of the difficulty you are having keeping up, they could bring prepared meals so you and your loved one both could eat earlier. If something like that would be helpful to you, don't be afraid to suggest it.

- **My uncle was cured with coconut oil.** You will hear fantastic stories of how other people were cured using some obscure medication or alternative product. Each person with Alzheimer's is unique and will react differently to drugs, supplements, or miracle cures. If you find something that seems to help, you should feel welcome to try it…or not. Some things may help slow the progression or appear to minimize symptoms, but at this point, there is no proven cure for Alzheimer's.

- **Of course Dad is too tired to attend big events, but my event is different.** Everyone says they understand the illness and how taxing daily activities are for the person with Alzheimer's and their main caregiver. This often changes when they are the ones holding an event. They think their event is somehow going to be different, easier, and more enjoyable for your loved one and you. Their wishing this will not make it so. Even if your loved one enjoys the occasion, these people will never recognize the struggle your loved one will experience later. They are thinking of themselves and not the best interests of your loved one.

- **Why can't you host our Christmas party?** Unless they also are caring for someone with Alzheimer's, few people can come close to imagining your daily challenges. The situation they glimpse appears so much easier to handle than the long, debilitating grind you are experiencing.

Comments like these are frustrating, if not infuriating, to hear and deal with. Trying to explain the situation to the offenders rarely helps. Few people, if any, will begin to understand and many will take your refusal to do what they want as a rejection or even an insult. One of the hardest things about Alzheimer's is learning you cannot please everybody.

Personally, it was easier for me to let comments like these go without any response at all. When I did try to explain, I wasn't heard. Listeners thought I was complaining or speaking unkindly of my husband. They were uncomfortable, and they didn't really want to know that anything was amiss.

I attended Catholic school as a small child. The nuns would tell us to offer the tough moments in our lives up for the poor souls in purgatory. This is a response well applied at times like this. Comments can seem so thoughtless and be very hurtful, but there is little to be done about it. When you can't change someone's understanding, just let it go. Let that be your prayer.

WHAT TO DO WHEN OUTSIDERS SAY THINGS THAT OFFEND OR UPSET YOU:

1. Ask whom they have cared for, for how long they offered that care, and how it went. If they have not cared for someone with Alzheimer's for a significant amount of time, just tune them out.

2. Remind yourself that they are not intentionally trying to hurt you. They simply cannot possibly understand what your life is like.

3. Let it go. Reasoning with thoughtless people can be no less difficult than reasoning with someone with dementia.

9.   Caregiving is Costly

WHAT IT'S LIKE

You quit your job three years ago so you could
provide necessary care for your ailing mother. You
checked the money you paid into social security
and realized not only are you not earning an
income anymore but are now missing making
payments into social security and a pension plan
that you will surely need yourself later in life.

WHAT I LEARNED

Whether we pay caregivers or give up our career to
care for our loved ones ourselves, providing care for
someone with Alzheimer's degrades our current and
future financial situation.

According to the Alzheimer's Association of America, Alzheimer's disease is the most expensive medical condition in the nation. In 2017, 15.5 million caregivers provided an estimated 18.2 billion hours of unpaid care valued at more than $230 billion. In addition, it is estimated that Alzheimer's and other dementias cost the nation $259 billion. By 2050 that price tag is expected to exceed $1 trillion.

Women are caught in the Alzheimer's circle at the highest rate because we are the majority of caregivers. Lost wages, the emotional impact of caring for someone with Alzheimer's, and the higher likelihood of developing the disease hits women the hardest. Our projected risk of developing the disease at age 65 is one in six compared to one in eleven for men.

Women typically receive only half as much in pension income as men, and two out of three women over 65 live alone—and on one income—in stark contrast to one in four men. Women are also 60% more likely to care for those with Alzheimer's without pay and therefore are not developing professionally or accruing pension and social security benefits during that time period. Depending on the number of years that a woman outlives her spouse or parent, she can end up in a financially dire position in her own senior years, primarily because of her willingness to provide care for a loved one with Alzheimer's.

The choice between providing care and hiring outside caregivers depends on our resources, our own ability to provide care, and the status of our career. The cost of hiring an outside caregiver will vary with their capabilities and experience—and it is critically important to hire a person who has experience working with dementia clients. Caring for someone with Alzheimer's is entirely different from caring for someone who is physically challenged.

Because of the mental, emotional, physical, and safety issues that must be addressed in caring for someone with Alzheimer's, such care comes with a higher price tag than caring for those needing physical assistance. Many Alzheimer's sufferers need both. Prices differ across the country, but in 2017 the national average for home health care averaged $20 an hour. Assisted living homes that offer memory care averaged $4,400 per month. However, this fee varies greatly in many areas. A $5,000 to 11,000 monthly charge is typical in many locations.

The cost to caregivers for their own health care is great as well. Family members who are caregivers to someone with Alzheimer's and other dementias had a $10.9 billion tab in additional health care costs themselves. More than half reported their stress level was "high" or "very high," and reported significantly more symptoms of depression than non-caregivers of similar ages, which typically adds a toxic effect on physical health. So in addition to loss of wages, pension, and social security, caregivers may experience significant medical expenses and diminish their ability to find work in the future.

Our family physician recommended hiring extra care when my husband Marshall was diagnosed. He also thought Marshall should have been admitted to a home several years earlier than he was. I thought I knew better than the doctor and cared for my husband alone for the first nine years of his disease. I wanted to capture the time with him while he remembered me and believed my care was best for him as well. I also wanted to delay the cost of help for as long as possible.

I saved hundreds of thousands of dollars in care costs and shared more time at home with Marshall, but overall my decision was foolish. Caring for my husband by myself created tremendous emotional and physical stress on my well-being. Not only did I lose earnings, I now suffer from several serious stress-related conditions that are at least long-term and may be permanent. Now my own medical care is costly and my physical condition may limit my physical abilities—and my potential to earn income—in the future.

If you should decide to care for your loved one, you may want to look into long-term care insurance for yourself. This will offer financial assistance in the now-more-likely event you will need care yourself someday.

You should also discuss with other family members the need for everyone to contribute toward your loved one's care. This is a very difficult discussion, one many want to delay or ignore. Yet caring for a parent, sibling, or spouse should not be the obligation of one person. All family members should do what they can. Everyone must step up to offer time or money to cover expenses.

When insurance and personal and family assets are depleted, public aid may be available. Contact local and public agencies early in the progress of the disease to discover what help your loved one may qualify for. A common misconception is that medical insurance will cover hired caregivers in our home or long-term care in an assisted living home. Medical insurance and Medicare only *contribute* toward doctor and hospital bills. They may cover short stays in assisted living facilities or skilled in-home services in some circumstances, but they *do not* cover the daily living assistance needed for most people with Alzheimer's.

Medicaid will cover the largest share of long-term care services in select facilities if your income level and savings fall below a certain level and other requirements are met. The rules regarding eligibility for Medicaid, in terms of income and resources, are complex. Most often, nearly all other assets (with the exception of your home) will have to be depleted before you qualify. Any pension or Social Security benefits that the person with Alzheimer's receives will be absorbed by Medicaid to supplement this care.

One last very important consideration is that our loved ones' legal affairs should be put in order at the onset of Alzheimer's, if they are not already arranged. It will be too late to take action in later stages of the disease. At that point, they will not be cognitively or legally able to execute these important documents and it then becomes more challenging for caregivers to assist them with their finances, legal obligations, and medical issues. Necessary documents include:

- Will
- Living trust
- Power of attorney for healthcare
- Power of attorney for property
- Access to savings and investments
- Control of medical and any long-term-care insurances

We also need to bring our own financial and legal documents up to date. Because of our loved ones' situation, we, of all people, should understand their importance. The time and expense required to draw up these legal documents will be well rewarded in the not-so-distant future.

....

WHAT TO DO WHEN FINANCIALLY STRESSED:

1. Ask family members to contribute either caregiving time or financial assistance. Do this on a regular basis.

2. Check local resources for care that is free, moderately priced, or charged on a sliding scale.

3. Inquire about public assistance

....

10. We Cannot Care for Our Loved Ones Alone

WHAT IT'S LIKE

You are wiping up the milk spilled inexplicably across the kitchen floor when you realize your wife has walked out the door. It's below zero outside and she isn't wearing a jacket.

WHAT I LEARNED

In later stages, additional help is required. Our loved ones need the care of an entire team.

Caregiving is rarely something we go into fully prepared. We inherit the responsibility because someone close to us needs our help. With Alzheimer's, our loved ones aren't even aware they need us, but our assistance is required, more so with each passing day.

That transition from spouse, sibling, or adult child to someone who eventually takes over our loved ones' entire lives usually comes at the price of mounting frustration on both sides. They don't want a guardian any more than we want to be one. But here we are, and in this relationship we are the only ones who can make sense of the situation. We already had an over-scheduled life, full of commitments and responsibilities, and now are acquiring more than double that.

The role of caregiver for a loved one with Alzheimer's brings with it an ever-progressive increase in responsibilities. As our loved ones' cognitive abilities decline, the list of things they need help with grows longer. A point will come when it will take several people—a team—to adequately care for them.

Researchers have described seven distinct stages of Alzheimer's. In the early stages, we may not even know our loved ones have the disease. As we begin to notice strange behavior, we may attribute it to other factors: normal aging, overwork, or stress. The way they act can be unsettling because we don't understand their changing behavior.

A diagnosis of Alzheimer's, as the disease progresses, clarifies the situation. Educating ourselves about the inevitable progress of the disease can help arm us to deal with it and prepare for the hardships ahead.

Certain distinct symptoms are commonly seen at each stage of the disease's progression. The early stages typically evolve over two to four years, middle stages from as little as two years up to a decade, and late stages generally last one to three years.

Common symptoms associated with each stage are:

1. **Normal Function:**
   The disease has taken hold but no symptoms are yet evident.

2. **Earliest Signs of Alzheimer's:**
   Very mild cognitive decline. Symptoms are not visible to friends and are probably not yet revealed in memory exams, but information is not as easily recalled as in the past.

3. **Early Stage Alzheimer's:**
   Mild cognitive decline. Our loved ones begin to have trouble remembering even familiar names and recalling new information. They misplace valuable objects and begin to have difficulty planning and organizing.

4. **Early-Mid Stage Alzheimer's:**
   Moderate cognitive decline. Mental arithmetic, managing finances, performing complex tasks, and recalling personal history grows more challenging. Inexplicable changes in mood become more common.

5. **Moderate or Mid-Stage Alzheimer's:**
   Moderately severe cognitive decline. Symptoms are distinctly noticeable. People with Alzheimer's now have greater difficulty recalling basic personal information, performing simple mental arithmetic, and choosing appropriate clothing. They are often confused about time or unable to recall the day of the week. They can remem-

ber significant personal details about themselves and still do not need assistance with eating or using the toilet.

6. **Moderately Severe Alzheimer's Disease:**
Severe cognitive decline. Memory and personality changes require more assistance with daily activities. Our loved ones are not always aware of their surroundings and may not recognize people dear to them, even a spouse. They are more restless at night. Some toileting assistance is often needed. They grow paranoid, suspicious, repetitive, and compulsive. They may wander in confusion.

7. **Severe or Late Stage Alzheimer's:**
Very severe cognitive decline. At this stage of the disease's progress, people with Alzheimer's struggle to carry on a simple conversation and control physical movements, including swallowing. Assistance with every facet of daily living activities is necessary around the clock.

Our loved ones' symptoms will not pigeonhole neatly into any one stage. Most likely we find that the behaviors we observe fit largely in one category with a few symptoms in surrounding stages. The assistance they require will increase as their needs change.

In the early stages, our loved ones may need a friend more than a caregiver. They will probably require support in keeping appointments, managing their finances, taking medications, and remembering names.

At this stage we want to encourage them to be as independent as possible. We are their safety net. We keep them on track. This is a good time for us to learn as much as possible about the disease and our changing role in caring for them.

Their ability to function independently becomes more of a challenge in the middle stages, and our own coping mechanisms will be sorely tested. We will be required to be increasingly patient. Maintaining simple and regular daily routines can help to keep both us and our loved ones calmer.

At this point, we have reached the time when we must closely observe our loved ones' actions and remove from their control some of the activities they can no longer adequately—or safely—do for themselves. There will be many difficult conversations over time as we take away their checkbook, their driver's license, their right to live independently, and their freedom to leave the house on their own.

In later stages, our assistance will be needed with everything they do. We have to plan ahead and think clearly for both them and us. We need to suggest activities that will hold their interest: listening to their favorite music, reading, looking through family photos, playing a basic game or solving a simple puzzle, taking a slow-paced walk. Such familiar activities help keep them occupied constructively and offer enjoyable moments we can share.

Since our loved ones may at some point be unaware whether they've eaten recently, it is important to monitor their food and liquid intake. We'll also want to assist them to the bathroom at regular intervals to prevent accidents. In later stages, people with Alzheimer's have incontinence issues because they don't realize they have to use the rest room, simply cannot find it, or don't even remember the process of going to the toilet. A regular schedule of bathroom visits will help minimize their incontinence.

Checking their overall physical health—their skin, hair, and teeth—so that they are clean and free of sores is very important. It's unlikely they will be aware of a problem themselves. We caregivers have to be on top of this so a developing condition does not become more severe.

The stress load can easily overwhelm us at this time. All attention is focused on the loved one, leaving little or nothing for us, the caregiver. Our loved ones may not always be kind or cooperative, and they will rarely be grateful. In fact, they will tend to resist our efforts. They believe nothing is wrong and therefore don't understand or accept that they need our help.

Living with someone with Alzheimer's can sometimes make us feel like we are living with someone from another planet. Our world grows more and more foreign to them and theirs to us. Objects, people, and language become unfamiliar and disturbing. And when our loved ones are disturbed, we too can grow agitated around them. Their thoughts, words, and actions are as unusual to us as ours are to them.

The statistics measuring the well-being of members of the family offering care for Alzheimer's sufferers are nothing less than alarming. The burden of the responsibilities we carry at this point becomes more extensive and our own resources become more depleted than those of caregivers helping someone with almost any other illness. More than 30% of caregivers of Alzheimer's victims die before the person they have been caring for.

For our own good, and for the good of our loved ones, we caregivers must take time for ourselves. We are less likely to react impatiently or make a mistake with their care if we are well rested. Spending time with friends—away from our loved ones—is essential to our well-being. Even taking a small, flexible part-time job or volunteer position can be helpful. Caregiving can be isolating, and when we are isolated our own health and well-being can begin to deteriorate. Immersion in community is critically important for our own health—mental, physical, and spiritual.

It's easy to burn-out when we are continually thinking for someone else as well as caring for his or her every emotional and physical need. The accumulation of stress hormones in our own systems will reduce our immune function with debilitating effects. And if we become seriously ill, we can no longer effectively care for our loved ones with Alzheimer's.

Chronic stress manifests itself in multiple mental and physical pathologies:

- Anxiety
- Depression
- Exhaustion
- Insomnia
- Muscle pain
- Depression
- Severe weight gain or loss
- High blood pressure
- Weakened immune system

It is critical for caregivers to take well-understood steps to avoid these problems ourselves. We must exercise, meet with friends, seek intellectual and cultural stimulation, meditate, visit a counselor, and simply be alone. It's necessary for our own mental health for us to periodically step out the door. We need breaks to rejuvenate. Our loved ones need us to care for ourselves.

And most likely, we still have to take ample time to attend to the other people and responsibilities in our life. We don't want to ignore everyone else in our circle. They are also people who mean much to us. We may even have another parent or family member in need of care, or children or grandchildren who need our time, love and attention.

Creating a team to care for our loved ones is the most critical step we can take in managing Alzheimer's. The more assistance they need, the more help we will need with their care. If we try to do everything alone, we are only setting ourselves up for failure. We will be overwhelmed and overtired. Pacing ourselves will allow us to succeed in caring for them to the best of our ability for a longer period of time.

Most often, we cannot count on family members and friends alone to provide the support we need and must hire professional caregivers. The decision to hire caregivers in the home comes with pros and cons, as all things do. When caregivers assist us with daily care, we are less tired and can enjoy more relaxing times with our loved ones. But introducing a stranger into the intimacy and privacy of our home brings with it its own problems. Necessary as it may be, it is still intrusive.

Before hiring someone, check each candidate's experience, training, and qualifications. A reputable agency can supply this information. Otherwise well-qualified caregivers with experience as companions and drivers for people in need of physical assistance are probably not adequately prepared to care for someone with Alzheimer's. If paid caregivers lack specific training and experience with this population, problems will undoubtedly arise. If our loved ones have long-term care insurance, the caregiver will be expected to meet the insurance company's qualifications and typically must be employed by an accredited agency.

Don't wait too long to explore options for help. It will take time to gain necessary approvals, and a 90-day waiting period before coverage begins is normal. Coverage varies by insurance company and by the age at which the insured acquired the policy. It commonly pays a daily maximum and will someday reach an ultimate total limit of coverage. Like a bank account from which funds are only drawn and never added, long-term care insurance can be quickly depleted.

I used a professional caregiving agency for my husband Marshall's in-home care. All of the caregivers were compassionate and efficient, but the ones who were not experienced in working with people with Alzheimer's made critical errors while caring for him. Because he appeared confident and capable, they weren't aware that Marshall required as much attention as he actually did.

We all are human and make mistakes. Even the best professional caregiver can overlook a potentially dangerous situation or miss something with a patient's care. You may have to try a few outside caregivers before settling on one or more who work well with you and your loved one. Think of the caregivers you let into your home as members of a team and consider how well you all work together.

As the disease progresses, more than one caregiver will be needed. This can make your home life chaotic if not managed well. The fewer people in and out of your home the better, but it isn't reasonable to demand that one person or a handful of helpers work unsustainable hours.

Asking other family members to help you may seem like asking for a personal favor, but remember that they will be helping their own loved one, not just you. Aren't we are all obligated to pitch in when someone we love is in need? However, enlisting help from other family members may not work for a variety of reasons. Many families are small and family members sometimes live too far away or are physically or emotionally unable to assist. Sometimes local organizations or faith communities can become a valuable resource. Many even provide excellent elder day care at a reasonable rate.

WHAT TO DO ABOUT GETTING ADDITIONAL HELP

1. Encourage family members to commit to caring for your loved one on a regular schedule.

2. Investigate qualifications, costs, and payment options of caregiving agencies.

3. Inquire about community organizations or faith communities that may offer senior care.

11. Assisted Living Is NOT Abandonment

WHAT IT'S LIKE

After months of denial, you finally admitted that you can no longer care for your sister at home. You accept her doctor's advice to place her in assisted living for memory care. Signing those admittance papers still made you feel as if you have abandoned her. For months, each time you leave the facility you walk away in tears.

WHAT I LEARNED

Moving our loved ones to an assisted living home is a heart-wrenching decision, but there will come a time when it is best for both us and them. We will remain an important, loving—and still dedicated—part of their lives.

We often hear people say they will never place their spouse or parent in a facility. They feel that would be deserting their loved one in their greatest hour of need. I felt that way for many years, but came to understand that such an impulse was born out of good intentions and lack of experience, not out of a clear-headed analysis of what was really going to be best for my husband.

Maybe it is true that there is no place like home, but caring for someone with late-stage Alzheimer's requires more time and energy than one person can reasonably hope to provide. Caring for our loved ones will never be easy, but in later stages of the disease 24/7 care is essential. We caregivers obviously cannot assist a loved one all day and all night long, day-after-day, year-after-year. Recruiting enough family members and friends to help is often impossible, and hiring trained help can cost more than full-time care in assisted living. Unless we can retain a dependable team to assist us in our home on a long-term basis, keeping someone with Alzheimer's there may be detrimental for both our own and our loved ones' health and safety.

I know this from experience. I encountered a series of personal health issues as a result of caring for my husband Marshall, several of which were serious, before I cried "uncle." I kept telling myself that my husband was happier at home than he could possibly be elsewhere, so I trudged on. With each passing day my patience withered and my own health declined. We finally hit a critical point when I was literally too ill to care for Marshall.

During Marshall's last year at home, we hired one caregiver a few hours each week, who worked well with Marshall and brought me much needed relief. But when it became clear that those few hours weren't enough and we had to start using multiple caregivers, life became extremely stressful for both Marshall and me. He was particularly disturbed by his evening caregivers.

He would grow increasingly agitated as the day progressed in anticipation of their arrival, which was as upsetting for me as it was for him. The arrangement turned out to be more disruptive and stressful than helpful.

Our doctors, seeing Marshall in his agitated condition, insisted it was time to move him to a home specializing in memory care. As his neurologist pointed out, "When a caregiver's health is compromised, that caregiver is no longer effective." He told me frankly that Marshall now needed more care and attention than one person could possibly manage alone. Marshall now required an around-the-clock team.

Finding an assisted living home for dementia took time and careful consideration. We are fortunate to have many excellent choices nearby, but making the final decision was still difficult. The home I chose is exclusively for Alzheimer's and related dementias. The entire staff is educated about the disease and handle residents capably. They are compassionate and upbeat. Rather than being stuck in a wing designated for those with dementia, as is common in homes that include regular assisted-living quarters, Marshall can roam the building and the beautiful gardens freely. Few residents are found sitting alone or sleeping. Most are actively involved in activities and visiting with friends and other residents.

Even though I finally came to accept that the move was necessary, signing the extensive admittance papers was exhausting and emotionally draining. I prayed very hard about the decision and believe I was lead to the best choice for Marshall. But still, the tremendous responsibility of making the right choice, and the unfairness of having to make one at all, was overwhelming to me.

When balancing the decision of caring for our loved ones at home or caring for our loved ones in an assisted-living facility, we must make an objective comparison between the level of care available in each place. We have to consider our own health and the limits of our abilities, the health and safety of our loved ones, and our declining ability to protect and control them in their spiraling decline. These are hard questions we need to ask ourselves as the disease progresses, and we have to answer them with unflinching honesty.

We tend to delay making the decision until a catastrophic event forces our hand. As much as we may need the help, moving loved ones out of their home is heart-wrenching. We put the decision off until it becomes unavoidable: they've taken a severe fall, endangered themselves by wandering away and getting lost, or their primary caregiver suffers a severe illness or death.

The reason for the delay may even stem from our own fragile egos. We have a difficult time believing anyone else could care for our loved ones as well as we will care for them in their own home. But when they reach a point where they no longer fully understand where they are or who we are, they will likely accept anyone who cares for them with tenderness and efficiency.

Before selecting a care facility, we should look closely at as many as we have time for, do some online research, and speak to the residents and their family members of the ones we are considering. The comfort and care of our loved ones is paramount, but we need to remember that we also must feel comfortable with the facility and its staff. We will be visiting often and must work well with the people who will be caring for our loved ones.

An optimum floor plan in a memory-care facility flows well, with no dead ends. The community is typically divided into smaller, manageable sections, each with its own kitchen, dining room, family room, laundry, and tub and shower rooms. Residents can mingle throughout the building, but smaller group settings allow for quieter, more peaceful meals and better rest.

Once we have made a preliminary decision on a home, we should make a few return visits at different times of the day before signing the papers. We can always move our loved ones out later if we are unhappy with the home, but doing so will be disruptive to them and force us to absorb multiple move-in fees.

Here is a comprehensive list of points to consider when investigating assisted living:

- Is the facility privately or publicly owned?

- What accreditation, awards, or citations has it received?

- What type of reputation does it have in the neighborhood? Ask neighbors, community agencies, and nearby church and club members if they've had experience there.

- What do local physicians know about it?

- Is the décor pleasing?

- Is the facility clean? Does it have a pleasant fragrance—not antiseptic or medical?

- Does the floor plan offer enough room for your loved one to walk?

- What conditions are other residents in? Are they active or mostly in wheelchairs and beds?

- What are the social opportunities? Are residents there on par mentally with your loved one?

- Does the home offer meaningful physical, intellectual, and spiritual activities?

- How far is the facility from your home? (This is particularly important if you plan to visit often.)

- Does it offer respite care? If so, trying it for a short stay before making a long-term commitment will be well worth the extra money and effort.

- How far is it from the nearest reputable hospital?

- Does the home have on-site nursing care?

- Are there doctors on call? Who are they, and what are their accreditations and reputations?

- How often do doctors visit residents?

- What certifications do staff members have? How are they trained?

- What is the resident-to-staff ratio and how does that compare to alternative facilities? How many caregivers are available per resident?

- How do they secure the privacy and safety of residents?

- What is the visitation policy?

- Is the facility able to care for your loved one through the end of their life, even if something should happen to you?

- Is the cost affordable?

- Do they accept long-term care insurance?

- Do they accept Medicaid? At some point government assistance may be necessary, even if you are able to pay initially.

When our loved ones are finally registered in a facility, how to inform them that they are moving to assisted living for memory care is something that should be given careful consideration by the family physician, present caregivers, and staff of the facility.

There is no one right way to cross this threshold. We may feel that we need to explain the move to our loved ones first, even if we know they cannot truly grasp what we are saying. Doing so is likely to result in anger and depression and outright attempts at refusal. The most common recommendation is to simply walk them in the door of the facility and leave quietly as they become involved in an activity. If you find it too difficult to do this yourself, consider having someone you trust take them there.

The first few days can be rough, but most assisted living residents do well after a short period of adjustment. They may continue to ask about going home. Marshall still does. Though they may not really remember "home," they can recognize that the place they find themselves in is not it. In all actuality, they never can go home again for two reasons. One, their sense of home often consists of a conglomeration of places in which they lived. It is a place that does not, nor ever did exist.

More significantly, since our loved one's ability to remember continues to diminish, they can't remember the comforts associated with their home. Sadly, they never can feel at home anywhere again. Marshall asked to go home when we were in the house we shared together for decades.

It's odd for spouses to live apart under any circumstance. I have found this concept difficult to grasp myself. I am married but do not have my husband with me. Even in Marshall's limited mental capacity, he realizes it too. There was a time when he told others we were divorced or that I was dead. He couldn't understand our relationship: how can we love each other but not live together?

A common practice for new residents in assisted-care facilities is to pack their personal belongings in anticipation of returning home or to ask staff and visitors repeatedly when they can leave. They naturally mourn the loss of the way things were, as we all do. Over time, however, they grow more comfortable and accept the fact that this is now their home. And they will ask to return to the facility after tiring when out, though they may still talk about someday going "home" with us as well.

Our impulse is to quiet our loved ones' thoughts because we want them to be happy and because it is so upsetting for us to hear about their sorrow, but they have every right and need to express their feelings. We can help by hearing them out and then trying to redirect their attention to something of interest at the present moment.

In many ways, the transition is more difficult for us than it is for them. So much of our attention has been focused on them, often for many years, and we now have to rethink everything we do without them. There can be a huge sense of loss, especially if they thrive in their new home, even though that is exactly what we want them to do. It is hard to feel we were so easily replaced by total strangers.

When Marshall first moved to assisted living, I felt as if I was mourning his death. I had to keep reminding myself he was alive, just not with me all the time. Family, friends, counseling, and the passage of time are helping me get through this ordeal, but I am surprised at how incredibly difficult it is.

The weight of responsibility on us caregivers is greatly relieved with our loved ones' placement in a home, but this does not mean we are no longer intimately involved in their lives. On top of regular visits, there will be phone calls to our loved ones, if they are able to talk, regular communication with caregivers and other staff members, doctors, and insurance companies. We also must monitor our loved ones' need for personal items and clothing. Speaking with staff when we visit and on the phone between visits is a subtle but important way to remind them we are highly aware of the quality of care they are providing. It might even be a good idea to volunteer to assist at the facility on a regular basis or to help with special events and outings.

After an adjustment period to this sudden disruption in their lives, most residents seem to thrive on the regular schedule. They tend to be happier and more at peace. There are fun and appropriate activities during the day, a floor plan that allows movement in a free and open setting, and healthy meals. We caregivers can find ourselves surprised at their enthusiastic participation in activities in which they previously showed no interest.

And now that they are in a secure, controlled environment, they may require less medication. Residents can safely roam all night, if they like. There are no stairs to fall down or doors to wander out of, and staff is up throughout the night to look after them, so medication to control these behaviors may not be necessary.

In most cases the move to assisted living is positive. Freed from the constant burden of caregiving, we have a better opportunity to enjoy the time we spend together when we do visit our loved ones. We can enjoy looking through photos, reading, or watching a program together without the responsibilities of full-time caregiving. Mostly, we can better enjoy being in each other's presence.

....

WHAT TO DO WHEN YOUR LOVED ONE MOVES INTO ASSISTED LIVING

1. Call and visit often, and on a regular schedule.

2. Keep in touch with staff members.

3. Regularly monitor your loved one's well-being in the home.

....

12. The Present Is a Gift

WHAT IT'S LIKE

One afternoon you and your husband of twenty years are enjoying a quiet moment alone together in his new residence. He takes your hand and tells you he is in love with you. He asks if you will marry him.

WHAT I LEARNED

When caring for someone so intensely, however great the strain, we can always find moments of intimacy. The majority of our day may be challenging, but there remain times of joy—with our loved ones and in other parts of our life—that we must take great care not to overlook.

The greatest lesson I can share about Alzheimer's is to embrace the present. It is the place where we can still find our loved ones and is a constant gift not to be ignored. No matter where we are on the Alzheimer's voyage, we must remain mindful of moments to treasure. If we aren't attentive to these gifts—and in our overwhelmed state there is a grave danger we won't be—we will not appreciate them until they are gone.

In the first years after my husband Marshall was diagnosed with Alzheimer's, we had some of the most loving times in our marriage. I worked hard to be tolerant and appreciated every expression of love and tenderness we shared. The more loving I became, the more Marshall followed suit.

One of our favorite activities was a daily walk. We both got some exercise and chatted about what we were seeing along the way. It was our uninterrupted, private time together, a time we both enjoyed and looked forward to each day.

Alzheimer's certainly is not a part of our relationship with our loved ones that we anticipated or would ever ask for. As caregivers, it is up to us to enjoy the time we do have with them, which might be months or years or even decades. We humans are not very good at recognizing what riches we possess until they are taken from us. With Alzheimer's, it is even more imperative for us to stop and give thanks for our many blessings before they slip away.

When in the presence of someone with Alzheimer's, we are required to slow our pace, which is beneficial for all of us. Our loved ones force us to stop, take a breath, and simply be with them in the moment. Everything else we think is so pressing on our to-do list can wait, or be left undone. Little is more important than that special, quiet time we have left with them. We really don't always need to be moving full speed ahead into the future. It's good to periodically stop and focus on what's right in front of us, here, now.

And there are bonuses to these momentary pauses with our loved ones. We often encounter some unexpected humor. People with Alzheimer's will say some of the funniest things, because they look at life from such a different perspective. For example, ninety-two-year-old Betty warned her sister Mary, five years her junior, not to sleep with men she doesn't know. Mary had never done anything sexually inappropriate her whole life, but she found her older sister's admonition hilarious and touching at the same time.

And since objects are often misplaced by Alzheimer's sufferers, we will find strange things in surprising spots, like the time I found my husband's hairpiece in the silverware drawer. It looked like the carcass of a dead animal splayed across our everyday silver and scared the heck out of me, but it did give me a good laugh.

Eventually, through all of our experiences and research, we caregivers become experts on Alzheimer's and the time and effort it requires. We can find reference resources at local homes for dementia and from abundant online resources. We can join support groups where we can share our stories and learn from others going through a similar experience. Ultimately we learn much from our own experience.

We will make enduring friendships with those we meet in support groups, other caregivers, staff members, and medical personnel who care for our loved ones. These are gentle, loving people who enrich our lives as well as the lives of those we care for. I know I'm deeply appreciative of so many people who have shown great kindness to Marshall and, no less, to me.

I have much to be thankful for. I'm sure you do too. The stress of Alzheimer's can overshadow the good things in our lives, but if we reflect on our situation the list of things to remain grateful for is long. You might want to make your own gratitude list, that perhaps will include some of the following:

- Smiles shared
- Warm hugs
- The opportunity to care for someone who has loved and cared for us
- Excellent medical guidance
- Compassionate caregivers
- Respite times for us to rejuvenate
- Stories we hadn't previously heard
- Quiet, gentle times to be near our loved ones
- Support and love of family and friends
- Our faith
- Faith communities
- Support agencies
- Bonds with others in similar caregiving roles
- A new understanding of Alzheimer's
- Unconditional love from our grandchildren and pets

Some of us may also have what I call "the gift of sweetness" that can remain in our relationship with our loved ones. Often, after they forget who we are, they continue to remember the emotional relationship we shared. Every day Marshall tells me he loves me and how much he wants to be with me. Once I walk out the door, however, I know he forgets I was with him and before long he is likely to lose all attachment to me. But today, I thank the Lord for a gentle, loving marriage and soak in Marshall's sweetness. I cherish those "I love yous" and him calling me "his Mary." I hold these gifts close to my heart.

Even when Marshall does forget me and our decades together, I hope we can continue in our friendship, and that he will be comfortable and at peace in my presence. Like old friends, we might share time together and a glass of lemonade, sour, and sweet, and satisfying. We can appreciate the sunshine on our faces or holiday decorations or a gentle pat on the hand.

Our story is not over. Marshall and I have an undetermined amount of time left together, and we have many paths yet to cross. I can't predict exactly how it all will progress or end. I can only take things as they come and deal with them one at a time.

We caregivers have to remind ourselves to keep our hearts open. Even amidst the turmoil of such a demanding situation, good things are always happening. There's no denying that most days are intensely stressful when we are caring for someone with Alzheimer's, but if we do the most we can for our loved ones every day, in the end, we will have no regrets. We'll know we gave them our all and, perhaps surprisingly, we will come to receive some incredible gifts—peace in knowing our loved ones were tenderly cared for, cherished moments that were meant only for us, and the discovery of our own great inner strength.

WHAT TO DO TO MAKE THE MOST OF YOUR TIME WITH YOUR LOVED ONE

1. Stop fussing. Capture the little moments of joy.

2. Find the humor in some of the craziness.

3. At the end of each day, count your many blessings.

Resources

Administration on Aging
330 Independence Ave., S.W.
Washington, DC 20201
1-202-619-0724
www.aoa.gov

Alzheimer's Association
225 North Michigan Avenue, 17th Floor
Chicago, IL 60601
1-800-272-3900
www.alz.org

Alzheimer's Disease Education and Referral Center (ADEAR)
PO Box 8250
Silver Spring, MD 20907
1-800-438-4380
www.alzheimers.org

Consumer Consortium on Assisted Living
www.ccal.org
703-533-8121

Alzheimer's Foundation of America (AFA)
322 8th Avenue, 7th Floor
New York, NY 10001
1-866-AFA-8484 (1-866-232-8484)
www.alzfdn.org

Caregiver Active Network
1130 Connecticut Ave NW
Suite 300
Washington D.C. 20036
202-454-3970
www.caregiver.action.org

Financial Planning Association (FPA)
Denver, CO; Washington, DC
1-800-322-4237
www.fpanet.org

Medicare Hotline
1-800-633-4227
www.medicare.gov

National Adult Day Services Association (NADSA)
1421 E. Broad Street
Suite 425
Fuquay Varina, NC 27526
877-745-1440
www.nadsa.org

National Association of Area Agencies on Aging (N4A)
1730 Rhode Island Avenue, NW, Suite 1200
Washington, DC 20036
1-202-872-0888
www.n4a.org

National Association of Professional Geriatric Care Managers (GCM)
3275 West Ina Road, Suite 130
Tucson, AZ 85741
1-520-881-8008
www.caremanager.org

National Eldercare Locator
1-800-677-1116
Eldercare.gov/eldercare.net/public/index.aspx

National Hospice and Palliative Care Organization (NHPCO)
1731 King St.
Alexandria, VA 22314
1-703-837-1500
www.nhpco.org

Social Security Administration
1-800-772-1213
www.ssa.gov

Glossary

Alzheimer's disease: a progressive form of dementia. Early symptoms include impaired memory, thought, and speech.

Amyloid: A hard, waxy deposit consisting of protein and polysaccharides that results from the degeneration of tissue.

Aphasia: Language disturbance either in verbal expression or the ability to make sense of what is said.

Apraxia: Difficulty with motor skills with no known cause. Involuntary movements, such as shuffling.

Agnosia: Inability to identify familiar objects.

Assisted Living for Memory Care: An environment that provides personal and medical support to those with memory disabilities.

Cognitive Impairment: Diminished cognition—thinking and reasoning.

Dementia: Deterioration of intellectual faculties, such as memory, concentration, and judgment resulting from a brain disorder or disease.

Memory Impairment: Diminished capacity to remember.

Plaques: Amyloid plaques are abnormal aggregations of tissue that consist of a protein called beta-amyloid found living between the nerve cells.

Tangles: Twisted fibers of a protein called "tau" that build up inside brain cells.

Bibliography

BOOKS

Bliss, Susan J. *We Will Be Healed.* Chicago, IL: ACTA Publications, 2006.

Broyles, J. Frank. *Coach Broyle's Playbook for Alzheimer's Caregivers.* Fayetteville, AR: University of Arkansas, 2006

Butler, M.D., Robert N. *Learning to Speak Alzheimer's.* New York: First Mariner Books, 2003.

Doyle, Mary K. *Young in the Spirit.* Geneva, IL: 3E Press, 2013.

Huey, Jo. *Alzheimer's Disease Help and Hope.* Alzheimer's Institute, New Orleans, 2001, 2008

Huey, Jo. *Don't Leave Momma Home with the Dog.* Bloomington, IN: Trafford Publishing, 2007

Leblanc, Gary Joseph. *Managing Alzheimer's and Dementia Behaviors.* Outskirts Press, 2013

Mace, M.A., Nancy L. and Peter V. Rabins, MD, MPH. *The 36-Hour Day.* New York: Wellness Central, 1999.

Petersen, Ronald. *Mayo Clinic on Alzheimer's Disease.* Rochester, MN: RosettaBooks, 2014

Simpson, Carol. *At the Heart of Alzheimer's.* Gaithersburg, MD: Manor Healthcare Corp, 1996

Snowdon, David. *Aging with Grace.* New York: Bantam Books, 2001.

Veney, Loretta Anne Woodward. *Being My Mom's Mom.* West Conshohocken, PA: Infinity Publishing, 2012

White, Laurie & Beth Spencer. *Moving a Relative with Memory Loss.* Santa Rosa, CA: Whisp Publications, 2000

VIDEO

Hoffman, Deborah. *Complaints of a Dutiful Daughter.* Women Make Movies, (1994). 462 Broadway Suite 500Z New York, NY 10013, www.wmm.com.

Acknowledgments

Proverbs says, "Commit your work to the Lord, and your plans will be established" (16:3). Caring for a loved one is definitely the Lord's work, so it is no surprise that the Lord surrounds us with people to help us.

Thank you to our family physician, Dr. Edward Ward, III and Marshall's neurologist, Dr. Steven Lekah, whose expertise, wisdom, and compassion helped us from the very beginning to navigate our way on our long voyage with Alzheimer's, as well as his new doctors, Dr. Malhotra and Dr. Thacker.

Also, thank you to Christina Beasley and the caregivers from Your Senior Caregiving Choice, especially my dear friend, Marla Shega, who was the first caregiver, other than me, to care for Marshall.

I'm also grateful for the many devoted caregivers and staff who care for Marshall in his assisted-living home. These people have not only been superb at caring for Marshall on every level, they've shown great kindness and compassion toward Marshall, me, and our family from the first moment we walked in the door. They carried me through the depression of separation from Marshall with unending tenderness and continue to be accessible as the journey continues.

Thank you to those who read an early draft of this book including Mary Jones, Pam Sebern, Erin Lukasiewicz, Lisa Kluge, Dr. Susan Holstein, Patricia Brewer, and Dr. Herbert Sohn. Their guidance was most helpful.

I'm also thankful for the kindness and expertise of the people at ACTA Publications and In Extenso Press. ACTA publisher Greg Pierce is not only an experienced, knowledgeable, and highly respected professional in the publishing industry, he is a compassionate and thoughtful friend. Thank you also to publisher Michael Coyne of In Extenso Press for his excellent editing and new friendship. I especially want to thank Patricia Lynch of Harvest Graphics for a cover and text design that masterfully captured the essence of my book.

These friends have my great appreciation: Doris Maloney, who cooked more food for me than one person could eat; counselor Pat Somers, who kept me on track; Mark and Susan Holstein, who always share not only their very dear friendship and understanding but their legal and emotional support as well; spiritual mentor and friend Sister Alexa Suelzer, SP; Dr. Thomas Carr and his staff; and my life-long friends Susan Kezios, Mary Ellen Collins, and Sally Thomas, my stepson, Marshall, and his wife Lisa, Arlene Kluge, Gail Gaboda, Susan Heitsch, Susan Shivers, Ken and Terri Mate, Bob Hoge, Cheryl and Tim Felix, and Chuck Romano, as well as so many others who reached out to me during my pneumonia and pleurisy and through Marshall's transition to assisted living. All their phone calls, text messages, visits, food, hugs, smiles, prayers, and strong shoulders were the cure that helped me heal.

Most of all, I am humbled by the gift of love and support of my precious family, especially my children Lisa, Erin, and Joseph; son-in-laws Mark and Steve; grandchildren Daniel, Tyler, Isabella, and Nathan; siblings and siblings-in-law John Michael and Lori, Patti and Parke, Margaret and Jimmy, and "little brother" Jimmy; my nieces and nephews; and my entire extended family.

God is good to me.

Also by Mary K. Doyle

FATIMA AT 100, FATIMA TODAY
Ten Steps to World Peace

HANS CHRISTIAN ANDERSEN
Illuminated by The Message

GRIEVING WITH MARY
Finding Comfort and Healing in Devotion
to the Mother of God

MENTORING HEROES
52 Fabulous Women's Paths to Success
and the Mentors Who Empowered Them

THE ROSARY PRAYER BY PRAYER
How and Why We Pray the Christ-Centered Rosary
of the Blessed Mother

SAINT THEODORA AND HER PROMISE TO GOD
The Story of Mother Theodore Guérin

SEVEN PRINCIPLES OF SAINTHOOD
Following Saint Mother Theodore Guérin

YOUNG IN THE SPIRIT
Spiritual Strengthening for Seniors and Caregivers

Available from booksellers or call 800-397-2282
www.actapublications.com

Also Available

THE ART OF PAUSING
Meditations for the Overworked and Overwhelmed
by Judith Valente, Brother Paul Quenon, and Michael Bever

COMFORT AND BE COMFORTED
Reflections for Caregivers
by Pat Samples

CONSTRUCTING A NEW NORMAL
Dealing Effectively with Losses Throughout Life
by Helen Reichert Lambin

HIDDEN PRESENCE
Twelve Blessings That Transformed Sorrow and Loss
compiled and edited by Gregory F. Augustine Pierce

MUSIC TO HEAL THE BODY AND THE SOUL
MUSIC TO SOOTHE THE SPIRIT
by Sheldon Cohen with the New Horizon Singers
and the Pacific Pops Orchestra

Available from booksellers or call 800-397-2282
www.actapublications.com